A Modern Look at Medicinal Cannabis

A look inside the medicinal realm of the cannabis plant and how it's helping to battle a long list of ailments ranging from neurological diseases, cancer, stress, anxiety and a myriad of other conditions.

Brett Wysocki

Table of Contents

Introduction **6**

As we navigate throughout this book, you'll
learn.. 10

The Endocannabinoid System (ECS).................. **11**

CB1 and CB2 Receptors.................................... **14**

The Cannabis Plant – Sativas, Indicas & Hybrids
.... **16**

Cannabis Indica..................................... 17

Cannabis Sativa.................................... 18

Hybrids 19

**Various Factors of Consideration & Things That
Can Affect Your Experience With Cannabis** **21**

Titration & Dosing 22

Delivery Method 22

Concentration 23

Tolerance... 23

Set & Setting 23

Pre-Existing Conditions 24

Cannabinoids **25**

Terpenes **27**

Why Terpenes Matter............................ 28

Opioids Vs Medicinal Cannabis **30**

Popular Cannabinoids....................................... **33**

THC... 33

CBD... 37

Delta 8 41

Cannabigerol (CBG) 43

Cannabinol (CBN) 45
Tetrahydrocannabivarin (THCV) 46
Cannabinoids Outro 47
Enter Medical Cannabis 49
Medicinal Cannabis – Ailments & Treatments ... 50
Some questions to consider 50
Alzheimer's Disease 52
How Cannabis Can Help 52
ADHD 56
How Cannabis Can Help 57
Epilepsy 58
How Cannabis Can Help 59
Parkinson's Disease 63
How Cannabis Can Help 65
Chron's Disease 68
How Cannabis Can Help 69
Multiple Sclerosis 71
How Cannabis Can Help 72
Insomnia 74
How Cannabis Can Help 76
Post-Traumatic Stress Disorder (PTSD) 80
How Cannabis Can Help 83
Nausea 87
How Cannabis Can Help 88
Anxiety and Depression 91
How Cannabis Can Help 93
Glaucoma 96
How Cannabis Can Help 97
PMS 100
How Cannabis Can Help 102
Arthritis 103
How Cannabis Can Help 105

Migraines...**108**
   How Cannabis Can Help.....................................109
Anorexia **112**
   How Cannabis Can Help.....................................114
Cancer...**117**
   How Cannabis Can Help.....................................119
Conclusion..**124**
Other Books By The Author................................**126**
One Last Thing… **127**
Works Cited **128**

Introduction

Cannabis is a subject that stirs up a lot of emotion and controversy among various social groups including doctors, scientists, researchers, politicians, religious groups and certainly the general public as a whole.

Despite the fact that cannabis is illegal under federal law, there are some states where it's been recreationally legal for years and it's quickly becoming legalized medically in a growing number of states.

Proponents claim that cannabis has proven to be effective in treating a variety of different ailments such as stress, depression, anxiety, insomnia, acute/chronic pain, arthritis, cancer, Parkinson's disease, PTSD, Crohn's Disease, Multiple Sclerosis, glaucoma, ADHD, Alzheimer's and opioid addiction just to name a few.

Adversaries wonder if its effectiveness has REALLY been proven ... Is it safe? Is it addictive? How is it helping these various conditions and at what cost?

Before diving into this book, it's important that as rational human beings we move forward with an open mind. Although ancient cultures have been using cannabis since 500 B.C. as an herbal medicine, people in the United States didn't start using cannabis for recreational purposes until the early 1900's. In fact, it's not until 1964 that we were able to isolate and characterize the main psychoactive ingredient of cannabis, THC, or Tetrahydrocannabinol.

We need to keep an open perspective while realizing that we still have much to learn about cannabis and its medicinal potential. As a matter of fact, for the last half century, the University of Mississippi has had the sole contract with the Federal Government of the United States to be the government's only provider of cannabis for research purposes.

As I write this book, cannabis researcher, Dr. Sue Sisley, is suing the U.S. Drug Enforcement Agency (DEA) and the Attorney General to be ordered to process the application to grow cannabis for clinical research. Sisley claims that the DEA has monopolized federally licensed cannabis research.

Because the federal government requires that researchers are only able to use cannabis from the University of Mississippi for studies, this limits researchers to low-grade cannabis in very limited varieties.

Sisley is quoted as saying, *"Scientists need access to options and we are handcuffed by a government-enforced monopoly that has only allowed me to study this really suboptimal study drug from Mississippi."*

Another important thing to keep in mind as we continue throughout this book is to reflect on similar patterns throughout history, such as prohibition. These examples reveal not only past misunderstandings, but also views, morals, politics and cultural stereotypes that helped to shape the opinions and viewpoints of cannabis in the past and present in society and culture.

Take for example, the 1980's, during the Reagan era. Nancy Reagan spearheaded the *"Just Say No"* campaign and paved the way for *"Above the Influence"* and programs like *D.A.R.E.*

Scare tactic commercials ensued, such as the infamous, *"This is your brain, and this is your brain on drugs,"* permeating the minds of those growing up at the time.

Additionally, this message seeped into the cultural fabric of the time through the influence of movie stars, tv shows and other forms of media inaccurately depicting the "dangers" of a plant they didn't quite understand or in fact know much about.

Cannabis remains federally illegal and is still considered a Schedule I drug.

According to DEA.Gov, a Schedule I drug is:

"Drugs, substances, or chemicals with no currently accepted medical use and a high potential for abuse."

Examples of other Schedule I drugs that appear alongside cannabis include:

- Heroin
- LSD
- Meth
- Ecstasy
- Peyote

I'm sure most people would agree that cannabis should be categorized much differently than some of the Schedule I drugs it's been associated with such as Heroin, LSD and Meth.

Please understand that no matter which "side" you think you are on when it comes to your stance on cannabis, that there still is much to learn about this fascinating plant.

Although cannabis has been around since at least 500 B.C., we've only just begun to learn more about it and it seems that we're finally starting to debunk a lot of its misconceptions. It's going to be very exciting learning more about many of the new medicinal properties and life enhancing benefits this plant may be able to provide us.

As we navigate throughout this book, you'll learn...

- *How cannabis works with our endocannabinoid system*
- *Cannabinoids and the difference between endo and phyto cannabinoids*
- *The different species of cannabis and their therapeutic effects*
- *Titration & dosing, delivery methods, concentrations & tolerance*
- *Set & Setting*
- *Terpenes*
- *The "Entourage Effect"*
- *Opioids vs. Medicinal Cannabis*
- *A few of the more popular cannabinoids*
- *Specific things to consider while using cannabis*
- *Specifically, how various diseases and ailments can be treated with medicinal cannabis*

The Endocannabinoid System (ECS)

Our Endocannabinoid System (ECS) is part of our neural communication network that helps our bodies to maintain homeostasis and it guides our mood and overall health. Apart from maintaining homeostasis, studies have shown that the ECS is responsible for repairing damaged cells without affecting our healthy cells, acting like a biological defense system.

It affects various different bodily functions such as appetite, memory, feelings of pain and even physical movement. Additionally, it also plays an important role in areas such as metabolism, immune function and reproductive function.

The ECS is the system that our body uses to process the pharmacological effects of cannabis.

The endocannabinoid system is present in all vertebrates which includes mammals, reptiles, fish, amphibians, birds, etc. and all of these vertebrates produce naturally occurring endocannabinoids. Plants on the other hand, produce Phyto cannabinoids, which can be seen as an example of the cannabinoids found in the cannabis plant which bind with CB1 and CB2 receptors in the human body.

Endocannabinoids are naturally occurring molecules that are produced by the human body, and were only recently discovered by scientists in the 1990's. This revealed a new signaling system comprised of cannabinoids and receptors.

Cannabinoids, which exist naturally in both humans and plants, work with our Endocannabinoid System to provide us various forms of natural relief. We are in the beginning stages of exploring the potential targeting abilities and fascinating opportunities we've yet to tap into with the endocannabinoid system.

Although initial research had suggested that endocannabinoid receptors were only present in the brain and nerves, scientists have since discovered that these receptors are present all throughout our bodies; our skin, fat tissue, pancreas, liver, skeletal muscles, heart, blood vessels, kidney, immune cells and our gastrointestinal tract.

Perhaps this is one of the reasons that cannabis is able to help treat such a variety of different conditions.

As we learn more about the endocannabinoid system, there seems to be growing promise due to pathological alterations of *cannabinoid signaling* that has been seen in various psychiatric disorders such as neurogenerative conditions like Alzheimer's and Parkinson's disease, as well as cardiovascular disorders, gastrointestinal disorders, multiple sclerosis, cancer and others.

CB1 and CB2 Receptors

The molecules in our endocannabinoid system that bind with the various chemical compounds in the cannabis plant, or cannabinoids, are the CB1 and CB2 receptors.

The CB1 receptors are mostly found in our central nervous system which is compromised of the spinal cord and the brain. These receptors are associated with cerebral and behavioral effects and directly play a role in memory, cognition, motor control, appetite stimulation, emotion and how we perceive pain.

When THC binds with CB1 receptors, it causes the CB1 receptors to "over activate" which in turn causes the psychoactive or elevated effects associated with THC.

The CB1 network, because of its important role in mediating our reward system, has huge implications for human behavior and it could offer us tremendous insight into human psychology and other diverse areas of study such as neurology, psychopharmacology, anxiety, mental health and other dependency related issues that are directly associated with the reward pathway system.

CB2 receptors are for the most part located in the peripheral nervous system and are directly associated with the immune system and inflammation response. Due to the fact that CB2 receptors are mostly concentrated within the body's periphery, it doesn't lead to any type of euphoric or intoxicating effects.

Activated CB2 receptors can help the body to promote relaxing effects and can even help to repair our bodies and reduce any feelings of pain without impairing our cognition.

When THC binds with CB2 receptors, it has shown a propensity to act as a potent anti-inflammatory that's extremely beneficial for treating conditions like arthritis, Crohn's disease and inflammatory bowel syndrome (IBS).

It's also used as an analgesic (pain killer) that has powerful pain-relieving properties. There is growing research surrounding CB2 receptors that aims at targeting pain management and countless other diseases and inflammatory issues.

The Cannabis Plant – Sativas, Indicas & Hybrids

The cannabis plant has been referred to by a variety of different names including marijuana, pot, weed, dope, Mary Jane, reefer, bud, grass, green, ganja, and surely many more.

Regardless, when most people hear any of the aforementioned terms, they usually mentally process thoughts associated with laziness, lack of ambition, or "pot heads" and "stoners."

But those who have been part of the cannabis culture for years know that cannabis is far more than that, in fact, it's much the contrary.

Currently as I write this book, according to various experts, there are 779 strains of marijuana. But, if you go on Leafly.com you'll see that they list thousands of different strains.

This number will certainly continue to change due to the fact that cannabis growers are able to manipulate the growth of their plants by cross breeding specific strains to create various hybrids based on the desirable effects and characteristics that growers are looking for.

There are 3 different species of cannabis:

1) Cannabis Indica
2) Cannabis Sativa
3) Cannabis Ruderalis
For the purposes of this book, you are going to learn more about the Indica, Sativa and Hybrid strains.

You'll learn which strains and subspecies are affiliated with different medicinal benefits and get a deeper understanding of medicinal cannabis.

Cannabis Indica

Indicas typically come from mountainous regions that have harsher climates and conditions. They tend to be shorter and bushier and develop thicker coats of resin as protection to their elements. Due to the shorter stature of the plant and their shorter flowering times, Indica plants are ideal for indoor growing.

Indica's focus their effects more on the body and are typically associated with feelings of sedation and relaxation. Because of this, Indicas are usually best enjoyed and preferred for night time use.

Therapeutic Effects That Indicas Produce:
- Promotes Relaxation & Reduces Stress
- Can relieve muscle spasms by relaxing your muscles
- Great for pain relief, inflammation, headaches, migraines & other acute pain
- Insomnia & other sleep related issues

- Reduces anxiety
- Nausea
- Can restore lost appetite
- Reduces frequency of seizures by acting as an anti-convulsant
- Assistance with those suffering from PTSD

Cannabis Sativa

Sativas typically come from areas closer to the equator and they thrive in temperate conditions. In contrast to their Indica counterparts, Sativa plants grow tall with narrow leaves and tend to have a longer growing season.

In contrast to Indicas, Sativas are associated with energizing and uplifting feelings. Sativas are used more for daytime use and primarily have a more cerebral effect as opposed to the body effects associated with Indicas.

Therapeutic Effects That Sativas Produce:

- Promote mental stimulation and provides uplifting & energetic feelings
- Increase sense of well-being
- Great for counteracting fatigue
- Helps patients who suffer with ADD/ADHD
- Increase your sense of focus
- Promotes creativity
- Can help to manage depression & elevate mood

- Offers relief from nausea, headaches & migraines
- Can help restore lost appetite

Hybrids

Hybrids are a combination of crossing Sativa and Indica plants, resulting in a strain that is usually either more Sativa or Indica dominant. Because of this, hybrids can have varying effects from both Indica and Sativa strains and they have become very beneficial in helping medicinal patients.

New strains are constantly being developed to help tackle specific ailments and medical conditions as well as to help enhance specific experiences for recreational users.

Therapeutic Effects That Hybrids Produce:

- Can provide a combination of both cerebral and body effects
- Provides feelings of relaxation
- Reduces feelings of stress
- Managing depression by helping to elevate mood
- Reduces anxiety
- Can help to restore lost appetite
- Can help with insomnia and lack of sleep

Please Note:

Hybrid strains can produce a wide variety of therapeutic effects in addition to some of the general effects listed above.

Various Factors of Consideration & Things That Can Affect Your Experience With Cannabis

At this point we now know, at a very basic level, the difference between Indicas, Sativas and Hybrids.

- Sativas are typically more cerebral and energizing
- Indicas are typically more sedative and relaxing
- Hybrids are a mix of both Indica and Sativa, usually dominant in one or the other (Ex.) – 60% Indica – 40% Sativa

But it's important to understand that this is not always the case. We all have a different biological make up, which means that we will all have a unique reaction as to how the cannabis will affects us. For the most part, with the majority of people, Sativas are more cerebral and energizing and Indicas are more sedative and relaxing. For some though, it could be the opposite.

This is where experimenting with different strains and *titration*, or controlling and measuring dosage, comes into play.

Titration & Dosing

You should always "Start low and go slow" until you start to understand how the cannabis affects your body uniquely and then begin to start learning how certain dosages affect you and begin to adjust to your most effective dose.

Delivery Method

Different delivery methods have different onset times, types of intensity and even elicit different feelings depending on how it was ingested into your body. For instance, smoking cannabis is delivered directly to your brain and usually has a fairly quick onset time, within a couple minutes.

In contrast, cannabis edibles can take anywhere up to 2 hours before onset as the delivery route requires it to be metabolized by the liver and usually results in a more potent type of high that lasts a little longer than the smoking route and produces a different feeling and experience.

Different types of delivery methods can include:

- Inhalation *(think vape cartridges, oils, crumble, shatter, rosin, etc.)*
- Nasal *(inhaling the product through a device with your nose)*
- Smoking Cannabis Flower *(the actual marijuana flower or "bud")*
- Oral *(edibles, capsules, etc.)*

- Sublingual *(tinctures, oral syringes, etc.)*
- Topical *(THC creams, CBD creams, sunscreens, etc.)*
- Suppository *(consuming cannabis rectally)*

Concentration

Simply put, how potent is the product? Are you smoking cannabis flower or are you using a concentrate? There are products out there that are pure THC distillate oils and there are products out there that are cut with cutting agents such as MCT oil and olive oil.

Tolerance

How often do you consume cannabis? If you've never or rarely ever consumed it, then you'll more than likely have a low tolerance. On the other hand, if you smoke every day or mostly use concentrates, you'll have a higher tolerance.

Set & Setting

What type of environment were you in? How much did you consume? Where were you? Who were you hanging out with? Did you receive any positive or negative news prior to consuming? What was your mood? Were you relaxed and happy or tense and anxious? Was this your first time or have you consumed before?

These are all important factors that can directly affect your experience.

Pre-Existing Conditions

PTSD? Parkinson's Disease? Multiple Sclerosis? Crohn's Disease? Glaucoma? Alzheimer's? Anxiety? Sleep issues? Depression?

Having an existing pre-condition plays a big part in determining which products and strains will be best suited for you. For instance, if you suffer from Parkinson's Disease, it would be more beneficial to recommend an Indica as it's a more "body" effect that is good for relaxing your muscles and it acts as an anti-convulsive.

But, if you were depressed, you'd be best to take a Sativa, providing you with uplifting feelings of happiness, euphoria and energy as opposed to an Indica that might induce a sedative and sleepy "couch lock" effect.

Cannabinoids

Cannabinoids as mentioned earlier in this book, exist naturally in both humans and plants, working with our body through the endocannabinoid system to provide our bodies a natural form of relief.

There are upward of a hundred different cannabinoids in the cannabis plant, but not all of them have been identified and this excludes cannabinoids we haven't discovered yet.

Although it's important to note that we are still in the early stages of what we're yet to learn about cannabis and its medicinal properties, there are a good number of cannabinoids that we do know about which produce a variety of different effects from anti-anxiety, muscle relaxing, anti-inflammatory, anti-bacterial, anti-fungal, promoting brain growth *(CBC – per University of Mississippi study)*, memory, suppressing or stimulating appetite and much more.

Although cannabis has a large number of different cannabinoids, most of them are present at very low levels. This will change as growers start to find ways to manipulate plants to yield higher levels of specific cannabinoids, which in turn could eventually create a variety of niche markets within the industry.

Terpenes

Terpenes are fragrant, organic compounds that are produced by flowers, plants and fruit. They have distinctive flavors such as berry, pine and citrus just to name a few.

Terpenes were originally developed in plants as a defense mechanism to repel predators and to attract pollinators. _The cannabis plant has naturally high levels of terpenes and each different strain produces different scents, flavors and effects._ They are secreted from the same glands that produce cannabinoids such as THC and CBD.

There are over 100 different terpenes that have been discovered in the cannabis plant and each strain has a unique terpene profile that can have unique effects to each person.

There are a variety of different circumstances that can influence the development of terpenes in the cannabis plant. Some of these different factors include the climate, weather, different fertilizers, the type of soil, amount of care the plant receives, among many others.

Individual terpenes each have their own unique effects ranging from things like relaxation, stress relief, focus, anti-anxiety and much, much more.

One example of a terpene is *limonene*, which is the essential oil of lemons and limes and is known to create effects associated with mood elevation and euphoria.

Cannabis strains that are high in limonene make a great choice for those suffering with anxiety and various forms of depression. Limonene also has antifungal and antibacterial effects which can make it a great choice for those with digestive issues.

Why Terpenes Matter

- They have medicinal benefits
- They provide the cannabis it's distinct flavor profile
- They directly affect the type of psychoactive effect or "high" the user experiences
- They contribute to the *"Entourage Effect"*

The ***"Entourage Effect"*** is where the various cannabinoids, terpenes and other compounds in the plant synergistically work together as a whole to produce a number of different medicinal and recreational effects/benefits.

This gives us an exciting look into the crazy potential of creating custom tailored strains that can act as medicine, create enjoyable recreational experiences and potentially alter the way we work and live.

Opioids Vs Medicinal Cannabis

Patients with chronic pain and those suffering from other pain related issues have more often than not, been prescribed treatments by their doctors that usually include some form of opioid such as fentanyl, morphine or hydrocodone to name a few.

These types of narcotics block pain messages sent by our peripheral nervous system by binding with receptors in our brain. Think of the opioid as a dam, but instead of blocking water it's blocking the pain messages being sent by our peripheral nervous system.

Although opioids can be extremely effective in managing pain, there are some extremely dangerous and negative down sides. Opioids are known to be highly addictive and often pose a high risk of overdose, which can be caused not only by taking too much of the medication but also by combining it with something such as alcohol, other medications or other substances that may cause fatal consequences.

According to drugabuse.gov, *drug overdose deaths that were caused by opioids rose from 8,048 in 1999 to 47,600 in 2017.*

Additionally, those that are coming off these medications are having terrible withdrawal symptoms ranging from insomnia, muscle pain, chills, and vomiting just to name a few.

Those who start relying too much on opioids could easily slip into an unwanted addiction. This starts to cause behaviors such as increased usage, more prescriptions and cravings for the drug.

Symptoms of opioid intoxication include:

- Constricted pupils
- Slow breathing
- Changes in heart rate
- Extreme fatigue
- Constipation
- Nausea

In a June 2017 study that was published in the journal *Cannabis and Cannabinoid Research*, they surveyed roughly around 3,000 opioid users. Cannabis was used as the control substance and the study measured the effectiveness of both opioids and cannabis for pain control.

In this study, 81% of the patients preferred cannabis alone and felt that it was a far more effective solution than even opioids and cannabis combined. Additionally, a staggering 97% claimed that the use of cannabis has helped them to decrease their opioid usage!

Furthermore, cannabis helps with various symptoms of withdrawals from those suffering from opioid addictions such as nausea and fatigue.

Popular Cannabinoids

Most people are familiar with marijuana's two most popular cannabinoids, THC and CBD. We'll also discuss a newer cannabinoid that is becoming increasingly popular with medicinal patients called Delta 8 and touch on a few other popular cannabinoids as well.

As we move forward in the book, I'll segment out and introduce specific conditions and then break down how cannabis can help those who suffer from these various conditions.

For the purposes of this chapter, we'll just briefly discuss some of the properties of cannabis, general benefits of medicinal marijuana and how it works with our bodies.

Let's start with the most popular cannabinoid associated with cannabis, THC.

THC

There has been a false narrative surrounding THC and cannabis, leading many to believe that CBD is the medicinal part of the cannabis plant and that THC is the intoxicant that people usually associate more with recreational use and getting "stoned" or "high." This simply is just not the whole story and it would be an injustice for people not to fully educate themselves before making such claims.

Before we can hopefully begin to change this narrative, we first need to understand what THC is, how it works with our bodies to produce its effects and how it can be used medicinally.

THC or tetrahydrocannabinol, is the main psychoactive ingredient found in the cannabis plant. It's scientifically referred to as "Delta 9," and like other cannabinoids, it acts much like the cannabinoid chemicals that are naturally produced by our bodies and binds to molecules in the brain's endocannabinoid system.

As THC binds with molecules in our endocannabinoid system, it's having a direct effect on our neural communication network in our body which regulates many different bodily functions such as mood, appetite, pain, memory and even physical movement.

Our CB1 receptors are mostly found in the brain and when THC binds with CB1 receptors, it causes them to "over-activate" which leads to the associated psychological effects or "high."

As mentioned earlier, THC can affect everybody differently and the way each strain affects our body is unique to each person.

But THC can also bind with CB2 receptors in other parts of our body such as those of the cells in our immune system. In this case, it can cause anti-inflammatory effects.

Additionally, THC has the chemical ability to increase dopamine levels. Dopamine is a chemical that acts as a messenger between brain cells and it directly plays a role in daily behaviors, attitude and outlook as it affects our mood.

Dopamine is associated with feelings of pleasure and satisfaction and it plays a major role in the motivational component of our reward system which motivates behavior.

This could lead to exciting work in the fields of human psychology and other areas of work such as neurology and mental health.

Medicinal Benefits of THC:

- Increased feelings of relaxation, elation and happiness which can help those suffering from daily stresses, depression and negative thinking patterns
- Certain strains can induce feelings of concentration and focus which is great for ADHD patients or those looking to aid their creative work
- Can increase appetite in those suffering from digestive disorders, eating disorders, nausea, and chemotherapy treatment

- Certain strains can produce an effect that induces temporary short-term memory, which is great for people who suffer from PTSD, depression and anxiety
- It can help to reduce pain by softening pain signals as they make their way to the brain
- Assist as a sleep aid *(typically this would be an Indica strain)*
- Creates elevated feelings of elation, euphoria and happiness *(typically a Sativa strain)*
- Has been linked to reducing aggression

There was a study done in the journal *Scientific Reports* which analyzed the data of over 3,300 medicinal marijuana patients who tracked their results with an app called "Releaf."

Over the course of almost two years (21 months), each subject would record the type of cannabis product consumed and its associated dosages and effects.

After nearly 20,000 recorded sessions, patients' symptoms improved by an average of 3.5 points based on an 11-point scale. The interesting part of this study was, that higher THC levels in the products consumed directly correlated with higher levels of relief that subjects received. This was not the case with CBD.

This is brought up not to take away from the many great medicinal benefits that CBD provides, but more to show that THC is not merely a recreational substance to get "high," but it's a molecule that has many beneficial properties that seem to be over-shadowed by outdated labels and by people who are inexperienced and uneducated on the subject matter.

CBD

It's seems as though CBD is gaining a lot of buzz in health and wellness recently and it's becoming a new trend in today's society. But with so much attention and discussion around CBD, it seems there's still a lot of confusion as to what it actually is, the benefits it provides and the difference be-tween hemp derived CBD and the CBD derived from the cannabis plant.

CBD or cannabidiol, is one of hundreds of differ-ent identified molecules found in hemp and canna-bis plants, just like THC. Often times people, in-cluding some budtenders, will describe CBD as the "non-psychoactive" part of the cannabis plant.

Although you may not feel "intoxicated" or "high," CBD does have a psychoactive effect as it directly interacts with our nervous system and can provide changes in our mood and behavior due to its anti-anxiety and anti-psychotic properties.

CBD works through multiple pathways in our body and it can interact with a variety of different receptor cells that can initiate a multitude of different physiological responses that help our body to promote homeostasis.

This makes CBD a good option for those who may have consumed too much THC, as CBD helps to balance you out and to decrease the "high" associated with THC.

So, although CBD won't get you "high," you can still benefit from its many therapeutic effects while maintaining a clear head.

When will I notice the effects?
CBD can take time before you truly start seeing effects and can take weeks of daily use to build up in our system prior to providing any results. In addition to that, it takes some experimenting in terms of dosages for each individual, as it will affect everyone uniquely. With that said, most experts agree that it's best to start with around 20-40 milligrams per day and to keep a journal and log results to help determine your proper dosage.

There are some desirable short-term effects that CBD can produce, such as that feeling of relaxation you get from smoking a high CBD flower such as *Harlequin GDP, which has a quick onset time* or something like CBD Nano-tinctures which can be done sublingually under your tongue.

Additionally, the anti-fungal and anti-inflammatory effects such as those in topical products like lotions and creams, can help to fight eczema and psoriasis.

CBD works great for a vast variety of conditions, such as but not limited those listed below:

- Acts as an anticonvulsant, becoming extremely promising for people suffering from seizures, tremors and epilepsy
- Anti-depressant
- Helps fight skin conditions such as eczema/psoriasis
- Has properties that can help relax your muscles
- Can help to prevent and treat neurological diseases such as Alzheimer's Disease, Parkinson's Disease and Multiple Sclerosis.
- Reduces inflammation
- Decreases anxiety
- Can help with those suffering from insomnia
- CBD can slow the progression of cancer cells
- May help to treat mood disorders
- Acts as a balance to THC's psychoactive effects

CBD - Hemp Vs Cannabis

The hemp plant is a close relative of the cannabis plant and both plants are members of the species cannabis, but you can think of them like cousins. Both plants produce extremely similar looks and smells which can be indistinguishable to those who are unfamiliar.

But there are some distinct differences.
CBD can be derived from both the Hemp plant and Cannabis plant.

Cannabis plants can contain THC percentages upwards of 30% while hemp plants will not contain anything more than .03% THC.

Due to the fact that it's essentially impossible to get "high" from the hemp plant, it's been made legal and hemp derived CBD can be found in drug stores, health stores and super markets everywhere in the country.

On the other hand, CBD rich medicinal cannabis is still illegal in the eyes of the federal government and it's only available to those in states with legalized medical or recreational use.

Due to the higher potencies, the CBD from the cannabis flower will be far more effective.

An easy way to think of it is to look at hemp as a supplement or a vitamin and to look at cannabis derived CBD as the medicine or pharmaceutical grade product.

Delta 8

Another newer and lesser known cannabinoid that is becoming increasing popular is *"Delta 8,"* which is a form of a mildly psychoactive cannabinoid. This is different from *"Delta 9,"* which is the most well-known psychoactive cannabinoid which produces the "high" people associate with the cannabis plant.

So, what is Delta 8?

It's similar to *Delta 9*, only it has much milder effects. It's been known to help with a variety of things such as mood, pain, memory and sleep. Additionally, studies have shown it to be 100% more effective than *Delta 9* for nausea and appetite which makes it great for those suffering from chemotherapy treatment and diseases such as Crohn's disease.

Delta 8 also boasts similar pain relieving and anti-inflammatory properties as that of CBD while producing a clear-headed, mild psychoactive effect that still allows you to stay productive and feel relaxed throughout the day.

It's great for those looking to battle anything from a mild headache to a painful migraine. Another great benefit of *Delta 8* is that you don't have to worry about the anxiety effects associated with consuming too much, like that of *Delta 9*.

Until recently, most clinical studies have been done on *Delta 9* and even more recently CBD, due to the recent explosion of CBD in health and wellness.

But there has not been much of a focus on *Delta 8*, a different type of psychoactive cannabinoid that we've only recently been able to isolate, which produces its own type of mild psychoactive effect and comes with its own set of therapeutic benefits.

If you're reading the eBook version, you can find more great information on *Delta 8* by visiting <u>this post on Trulieve's blog</u>.

The blog post referred to above, mentions at one point, an experiment that was conducted by government researchers in 1974 to test the effects of *Delta 8* on the immune system of mice.

During this study, *the experiment revealed that the cannabinoid Delta 8 had cancer killing abilities.*

Although you'd think this exciting news would provoke more press and continued research, the public remains generally unaware for the most part and it's taken the government decades to actually admit that *Delta 8* has the abilities to kill cancer cells.

The blog post also mentions a report that was conducted by the National Cancer Institute. <u>The report showed that Delta-8, Delta-9 and CBD were ALL shown to possess the ability to stop the growth of tumors.</u>

So, for a quick recap, Delta 8:

- Produces a milder, clearer headed high
- It helps with mood, memory, pain and sleep
- It's shown to possess the ability to stop tumor growth
- It's 100% more effective for nausea and appetite than *Delta 9*
- It has similar analgesic and anti-inflammatory properties as that of CBD
- It's a great solution for both a mild headache or a painful migraine
- Promotes a relaxing experience and is great for use throughout the day

Cannabigerol (CBG)

Cannabigerol or CBG, is a non-psychoactive cannabinoid that has sometimes been referred to as a "stem cell" for other cannabinoids and it can even be a precursor to THC or CBD. It has muscle relaxing effects and it can also be great for treating anxiety.

An article on <u>leafly.com</u>, shows many of the following medicinal uses and benefits that CBG has been linked to including:

- CBG reduces intraocular pressure, which is extremely helpful for glaucoma patients. This is due to a high prevalence of endocannabinoid receptors in our eyes.
- In a study dating back to 2015, CBG was shown to protect the neurons of mice that had Huntington's Disease (a fatal genetic disorder which leads to the progressive breakdown of nerve cells in the brain).
- CBG has anti-bacterial properties and is especially effective against MRSA
- In a 2017 study, a form of purified CBG was isolated from Delta-9 THC and was proven to be an extremely effective appetite stimulant for rats. This proves to be promising especially for patients that have anorexia, deteriorating muscle, severe weight loss, late stage cancer patients and various other diseases.
- CBG has been linked to inhibiting muscle contractions relating to the bladder which may help to treat various forms of bladder dysfunction and disorders.

There is a lot of promising and exciting research being done regarding the use and effects of CBG. This opens up a wide range of potential, especially as we learn more about how it interacts with other cannabinoids.

Cannabinol (CBN)

Cannabinol or CBN, is a non-psychoactive cannabinoid that is typically only found in trace amounts in cannabis and it forms when THC reacts with oxygen. Because of this, the longer cannabis is exposed to air, the more CBN it will likely have, up to a certain point.

Some of the potential benefits of CBN include…
Anti-bacterial:
In lab settings, research has shown CBN to be particularly efficient in fighting bacteria such as MRSA, which can sometimes be resistant to traditional antibiotics. This gives hope that perhaps further research can lead us to possible treatments with CBN being used as a proficient alternative to fighting various other bacterial diseases.

Neuroprotectant:
In a study using mice, researchers treated subjects that were affected with ALS, with doses of CBN. The study found that CBN was able to delay the onset of the condition and although more human studies need to be done, this gives us hope for the promise of cannabinoids to help battle various neurogenerative conditions.

Appetite Stimulator:
In studies using rats, increased CBN correlated with the amount of food the rats ate. Again, more human studies need to be done, but there is

evidence that suggests that CBN could be a good alternative for those looking to stimulate their appetite without the associated effects of getting "high." This could be promising for a variety of different eating disorders, people suffering from chemotherapy, deteriorating muscle conditions, severe weight loss, etc.

Glaucoma:
Studies have shown CBN to be effective in reducing intraocular pressure, which is one of the biggest risk factors for glaucoma.

Anti-Inflammatory:
CBN shows promise in fighting debilitating conditions such as rheumatoid arthritis and in some cases, it's shown to reduce occurrences of arthritis.

Tetrahydrocannabivarin (THCV)

Tetrahydrocannabivarin or THCV, is a psychoactive cannabinoid that actually suppresses hunger as opposed to stimulating it. This makes THCV a very interesting cannabinoid in terms of research for weight loss and diabetes.

Additionally, THCV has shown promise for:

- Reducing panic attacks
- Helping to improve tremors, motor control and brain lesions associated with Alzheimer's disease

- Stimulate the growth of new bone cells which has researchers interested to find out if it could be a possible treatment for those with conditions such as osteoporosis and other bone related issues.

Just like CBN, THCV is usually only found in trace amounts in the cannabis plant which can make it difficult to really obtain for those seeking it out for its possible therapeutic effects.

Cannabinoids Outro

There are dozens and perhaps upwards of hundreds of cannabinoids that we currently know about and this book will obviously not cover them all. The examples provided above were selected to show a small sample size of possibilities regarding the promising research being done on various cannabinoids and how they interact with our endocannabinoid system.

This all points to a future of a "Cannabinoid Commodity" market. As cannabis continues to become legal in various states and eventually at the federal level, you'll start to see more research done on specific cannabinoids.

Just like there are people who seek out higher amounts of THC and CBD respectively, you will start to see a migration towards niche markets opening up in the cannabis space that will target specific cannabinoids that are known for their specific therapeutic benefits. You can see this trend currently being played out with CBD.

For more information on additional cannabinoids, you can check out this great link below:

Leafly: List of Major Cannabinoids in Cannabis and Their Effects

Enter Medical Cannabis...

As mentioned earlier in this book, medicinal cannabis has been used to treat numerous conditions and ailments.

Some of these include:
Parkinson's Disease
Alzheimer's
General Pain
Arthritis
Depression, Anxiety, Stress
Loss of appetite
Crohn's Disease
Cancer
Insomnia
PTSD
Nausea
Multiple Sclerosis
Muscle Spasms
Epilepsy
ADHD
PMS
Anorexia
Glaucoma
Migraines

Medicinal Cannabis – Ailments & Treatments

Moving forward, we'll go over a long list of various ailments and how medical cannabis is helping to treat these conditions.

It's important to keep in mind that there are plenty of variables to consider, some of which we've briefly touched on, before deciding on your best method of cannabis treatment.

Some questions to consider...

- What specific condition are you looking to treat?
- What is the desired effect your looking for?
- Am I using this product while I work?
- Do I need something for a headache? Or do I have body pain?
- Will I be consuming this during the daytime or the evening?
- Do I have any pre-existing conditions to consider?
- If I don't want to smoke cannabis, is there another effective way I can consume it?

Medicinal cannabis has become increasingly popular and has been touted as a miracle drug, with many believing that it's reshaping medicine. It's hard to keep from being excited while realizing how early we are in our understanding about medicinal cannabis and how its already effectively treating many ailments such as the following:

Alzheimer's Disease

Alzheimer's disease is a terrible, irreversible brain disorder that has mind deteriorating effects such as destroying memory, cognition and the inability to perform the simplest of everyday tasks.

There comes a point where this disease will completely take over the mind and unfortunately leave patient's unable to take care of themselves.

With no cure and no current way to stop the progression of this awful disease, patients are looking for the best forms of treatment for symptoms and anything to help slow it down.

Severe symptoms of Alzheimer's include:

- Disorientation
- Memory loss
- Constant confusion
- Not being able to recognize friends and family
- Mood changes
- Aggression
- Agitation
- Sleeplessness

How Cannabis Can Help

Research suggests that cannabinoids may be helpful in stopping the buildup of amyloid plaques, which are found in the brains of Alzheimer's patients.

High levels of amyloid plaque can lead to clumping of these proteins which begin to build between brain neurons which in turn disrupts the cell function in the brain.

Cannabinoids such as THC, CBD and CBG have shown to be effective in helping to prevent cell death and the possible stimulation of cell growth in areas of the brain that are correlated with memory.

Additionally, cannabis can help to treat other symptoms associated with Alzheimer's disease such as depression, mood, anxiety, irritability and changes in appetite among others.

For instance, certain Sativa strains not only have the ability to alter mood with their happy and euphoric effects, but they can also increase energy, which is a great combination for those suffering from depression.

Also, some Alzheimer's patients can sometimes begin eating less due to changes in appetite and many cannabis strains can increase appetite and bring back the pleasure of eating.

A PubMed.gov study set to research the potential therapeutic effects of Delta 9 THC regarding the possibility of slowing or stopping the main characteristics of Alzheimer's disease.

The study also tested to determine if in fact multiple treatments were beneficial to subjects.

Listed below are the results of the study:
"We did discover that THC directly interacts with Aβ peptide, thereby inhibiting aggregation.

Furthermore, THC was effective at lowering both total GSK-3β levels and phosphorylated GSK-3β in a dose-dependent manner at low concentrations.

At the treatment concentrations, no toxicity was observed and the CB1 receptor was not significantly upregulated.

Additionally, low doses of THC can enhance mitochondria function and does not inhibit melatonin's enhancement of mitochondria function.

These sets of data strongly suggest that THC could be a potential therapeutic treatment option for Alzheimer's disease through multiple functions and pathways."

Although there is still much research to be done, there are some amazing results occurring with real people, such as this recent Forbes article featuring Greg Spier, whose father, a WWII vet, developed Alzheimer's.

After the onset of Alzheimer's, Greg's father began suffering from past trauma and suppressed terrifying experiences from the war, such as being in concentration camps. After working with doctors and seemingly exhausting all options, Greg's father found solace from his suffering through a CBD gummy that a family member "smuggled" him.

The article states:
"The effects were immediate and notable. As Spier recalls, his father became calm, slept well and the next day was more relaxed and lucid than he had been for months."

Apart from all the early research, it's stories like these that give promise and promote a positive outlook on the medicinal future of cannabis and the effects it may have in treating neurogenerative conditions such as Alzheimer's disease.

ADHD

There are a few different forms of ADHD, which stands for Attention Deficit Hyperactivity Disorder. People who suffer from ADHD typically suffer from symptoms such as the inability to stay focused, being easily distracted, forgetful and disorganized.

Currently, ADHD is being treated with medications such as Ritalin and Adderall. Both of these are stimulants and have been abused by teens, who have been reported in some cases to go as far as faking symptoms in order to get prescriptions.

Often times these are students who are getting them from friends, in order to help them with school and to perform better during big exams.

Ritalin, which is also known as *methylphenidate*, is labeled by the DEA as a ***Schedule II narcotic***, which puts it in the same class of drugs such as cocaine, morphine and amphetamines.

Adderall, which is combination of 2 different stimulants, amphetamine and dextroamphetamine, *is also listed as a Schedule II*.

Adderall works by increasing levels of dopamine which in turn stimulates the brain and is used to help increase levels of focus and concentration.

Common negative side effects that have been linked to both these drugs include:

- Nervousness
- High blood pressure
- Insomnia
- Decreased appetite
- Abuse

How Cannabis Can Help

Cannabis is also extremely effective at increasing dopamine levels, which in turn can help to combat ADHD by helping those who suffer with this disorder to better focus and concentrate on tasks at hand.

Cannabis Sativa strains can act as excellent examples of energetic, cerebral stimulants which can help to increase focus and concentration in users. An example of such a strain is the strain known as *"Green Crack."*

Users of this strain have reported a sharp increase in energy and focus, with an exhilarating mental buzz. In addition, this strain can have beneficial side effects that help to combat fatigue, stress and depression.

Epilepsy

According to HealthLine.com, it's currently estimated that *3.4 million people in the United States
suffer from epilepsy and 1 in 26 people will develop epilepsy at some point during their lifetime.*

Epilepsy is a neurological disorder that's known
for its recurrent, unpredictable seizures. It causes a
surge of electrical activity in the brain which leads
to a disruption in messages being sent from the
brain to other parts of the body.

Although the cause of epilepsy is not very clear,
it's presumed that it can be a result of severe brain
trauma, disease and family history.

**Epilepsy seizures can be categorized by (3) dif-
ferent types:**
Focal Onset
Generalized
Unknown Onset

Focal Onset:
Focal onset seizures affect one area on one side of
the brain and approximately 60% of all seizures
are classified as focal onset.

A person suffering from a focal onset seizure may
be awake and aware as to what's happening. This

type of seizure usually lasts a minute or two in duration and symptoms can be mild enough that those who suffer are able to work through them.

Generalized Seizures:
Generalized seizures affect both sides of the brain at the same time and more than 30% of people who suffer with epilepsy will experience generalized seizures. Sometimes generalized seizures can begin as focal onset and turn into a generalized seizure.

These types of seizures are often associated with loss of consciousness and sever muscle contractions.

Unknown Onset:
As the name accurately depicts, the origins of these types of seizures are unknown and they have sometimes been known to recur in clusters.

Symptoms of both focal and general onset can include jerking movements associated with the motor system, weak/limp or rigid/tense muscles or muscles spasms and twitching.

How Cannabis Can Help

Epilepsy often affects those who suffer from the disease in a multitude of different ways as often times those battling epilepsy are more susceptible to depression, anxiety and sleep problems just to name a few.

High CBD strains of cannabis have been linked to reduce the frequency of seizures and research suggests great promise in the use of medicinal cannabis for the treatment of epilepsy.

A report on <u>ScienceDirect.com</u> titled, *"Report of a parent survey of cannabidiol-enriched cannabis use in pediatric treatment-resistant epilepsy,"* is a survey that was done which aimed at targeting specific patients to include in a study exploring the use of high CBD cannabis in children with treatment-resistant epilepsy.

In this survey, 19 responses met the targeting criteria, in which all were children with treatment-resistant epilepsy.

Out of these 19 children:
13 children had Dravet Syndrome, which is a type of epilepsy with seizures that are often triggered by hot temperatures or fever often beginning around the age of six months.

4 children had Doose Syndrome, which is a type of epilepsy of early childhood often appearing between ages 1-5, which usually is accompanied by generalized seizures.

1 child had Lennox-Gastaut Syndrome, which is a rare and complex form of severe childhood-onset epilepsy.

1 child had Idiopathic Epilepsy, which is a group of various epileptic disorders believed to be strongly tied to genetics.

Prior to this study, the average number of antiepileptic drugs that EACH patient tried before using CBD was 12.

What the results of the CBD trials yielded:

- *84% of children (16 of 19), reported a reduction in seizure frequency while taking CBD*
- *11% (2 of 19), reported to be completely free of seizures*
- *42% (8 of 19), reported to see an 80% reduction in the frequency of their seizures*
- *32% (6 of 19), reported seizure reductions anywhere from 25-60%*

In addition to the numbers above, there were other beneficial factors or positive side effects that resulted from the use of CBD.

Some of these various effects included an increased sense of alertness, better overall mood and an improvement in sleep. Additional side effects included feeling drowsy and fatigued.

Overall, the results from the survey are very interesting and show promise in helping to treat severe forms of childhood epilepsy, seizures and help aid those with neurodevelopmental issues.

Parkinson's Disease

According to Parkinson.org, *nearly 1 Million people in the US will be living with Parkinson's Disease by 2020.*

This is a progressive neurological disorder that causes a loss of dopamine-producing neurons in areas of the brain that are responsible for our coordination and body movement.

Brain cells that produce dopamine, a neurotransmitter which is responsible for sending messages throughout the body that are associated with movement, begin to become damaged and start dying. This leads to various different movement issues such as lack of facial expression, inability to balance and muscle stiffness.

Symptoms for Parkinson's usually begin after about 80% of these neurons die.
These symptoms can appear very slowly and sometimes go unnoticed in the early stages of the disease.

There are a wide range of varying symptoms, but some of them include:

- Slowed movement
- Rigid muscles

- Impaired balance
- Changes in speech or writing
- Difficulty performing unconscious movements

The symptoms begin usually by affecting one side of the body but as the disease begins progressing, both sides of the body can become affected.

Patient's begin to lose their coordination and start getting tremors, which makes daily activities such as getting dressed in the morning, walking, eating, etc... increasingly difficult.

As the disease progressively gets worse and enters the latter stages, most patients will need full time care.

Current treatment of Parkinson's:
Currently, Parkinson's patients have treatment options such as medications that are used to replenish dopamine levels, which can improve coordination and help to stop tremors.

There are also surgical options such as implantable brain stimulators which identify the area of the brain that is malfunctioning and react by sending electrical impulses to the affected area, which can improve coordination and tremors in patients as well.

How Cannabis Can Help

Cannabis has long been known to have the ability to reduce tremors and it's even been prescribed by doctors dating back to the nineteenth century, who would generally prescribe it to their patients in the form of tinctures.

By binding with the CB1 receptors in the brain, cannabinoids from the cannabis plant have shown to improve coordination and motor ability in those suffering with Parkinson's disease.

Additionally, there have been studies suggesting that the neuroprotective properties from the cannabis plant may even help to prevent brain cells from dying and also prevent the buildup of the neurotoxins that are associated with the disease.

Cannabis has also been linked to helping patients with related side effects of Parkinson's Disease such as depression. Certain strains of cannabis can help to promote happy and positive outlooks, while increasing mood and energy.

CBD & Parkinson's:
An article titled, *"CBD: A Natural Remedy that Decreases Symptomatic Behaviors of Parkinson's Disease,"* on DementiaCareCentral.com, features work on the effects of CBD and Parkinson's Disease by researchers Alyssa S. Laun and Zhao-Hui Song from the University of Louisville.

They found that CBD acts as an "inverse agonist" on a receptor known as CPR6 which are found predominantly in a specific region of the brain associated with the connection of the cerebral cortex and the brainstem, which drive functions in our bodies related to movement, learning and emotion.

According to their research...
"Cannabinoid receptors run throughout our body as part of the endocannabinoid system regulating physiological operations including hunger, pain sensitivity, temperament, and memory. These natural receptors are affected in patients with Parkinson's Disease. As analyses continue, CDB is demonstrating relief for tremors, psychosis, and problems sleeping. CBD may also reduce depression and anxiety, and relieve pain. A study at the Colorado School of Medicine has demonstrated relief of issues including tremors and difficulty sleeping. CBD studies are also showing it as effective in treating the psychosis that comes with PDD (Parkinson's disease dementia). So far, patients are tolerant of low doses of CBD oil and report positive effects."

CBD has been shown in studies to be deemed as safe and well tolerated in those who use it and there has been no evidence on any abuse or addiction to CBD.

With that being said, there are a few potential, non-serious, side effects that may occur such as appetite change, feeling tired or diarrhea.

Chron's Disease

Chron's disease is an inflammatory bowel disease that affects the digestive tract by causing inflammation which can lead to abdominal pain, severe diarrhea, weight loss, malnutrition and fatigue just to name a few.

That being said, different areas of the digestive tract can be affected in different people.

Typically, in a normal functioning gastrointestinal tract, there are "good bacteria" that help aid us with digestion and our immune system knows not to attack these bacteria.

In those who suffer with Crohn's Disease, these same "good bacteria" are seen as invaders by our immune system and it responds by inducing inflammation.

At a certain point, people with Crohn's will experience chronic inflammation which can lead to:

- Extreme diarrhea
- Blood in stool
- Abdominal cramps
- Pain
- Frequent bathroom use
- Loss of appetite
- Fatigue

- Low energy levels

This chronic onset of Chron's Disease can have dramatic effects on the lives of those who suffer.

More often than not, feelings of isolation, embarrassment and worry can occur as there is a constant need to be near a bathroom. This leads to stress and it can especially carry over to the work place and other social environments as flare ups are unpredictable and can happen suddenly.

Current treatment of Crohn's Disease:
Although there is no cure for Crohn's Disease, patients have looked for relief through a variety of different treatments and medications including anti-inflammatory drugs, corticosteroids, antibiotics, immune system modifiers and a multitude of different nutritional supplements.

How Cannabis Can Help

Cannabis has been shown to be a great way for Crohn's patients to help alleviate some of their most disruptive symptoms.

In fact, medical cannabis is known for its anti-inflammatory properties and it's been shown to be extremely effective in a variety of other symptoms related to Crohn's such as:

- Reducing pain
- Lowering anxiety

- Calming nausea
- Increasing appetite

Essentially, what happens when these Crohn's patients start using cannabis, is that the cannabinoids from the plant help the body's immune system by stopping it from attacking the healthy tissue, while simultaneously providing pain relief and helping to increase appetite.

Although evidence regarding the direct relationship between cannabis and Crohn's is only anecdotal at this point, it's seen as extremely promising and encouraging. There are some patients who claim that it's even helped them to go in remission.

Multiple Sclerosis

Multiple Sclerosis is a chronic degenerative disease which causes the immune system to go berserk.

There is a fatty like substance that surrounds and protects our nerve fibers called myelin. In patients with MS, their immune system causes inflammation that damages or sometimes destroys this myelin which can alter or stop messages within the central nervous system, leading to a variety of neurological symptoms.

Symptoms can include the following:

- Numbness or tingling in the face, body or extremities
- Speech impairment
- Fatigue and weakness
- Muscle Spasms
- Depression
- Dizziness
- Impairment of muscular coordination
- Blurred vision
- Severe fatigue

Other less common symptoms can include:

- Tremors
- Difficulty swallowing

- Breathing issues
- Seizures

Current treatment of Multiple Sclerosis:

MS currently has no cure and there are only treatments that are sought after by patients with the goal of controlling the symptoms.

Most commonly, MS patients are prescribed drugs such as corticosteroids which can help to reduce inflammation and suppress the immune system in a way that helps to prevent it from attacking healthy tissue.

These drugs can be consumed by the body through multiple different routes including injections, orally or administered by IV (intravenously). Additionally, many patients use a consistent physical therapy regimen that can help to restore coordination and re-gain strength in muscles.

MS patients have also been known to use alternative methods to help combat their symptoms such as increasing their vitamin D intake, taking up yoga, acupuncture, meditation, relaxation practices and other forms of herbal medicines.

How Cannabis Can Help

The cannabis plant has dozens of chemicals that can have various effects on our mind and body, which as we already know works naturally with our endocannabinoid system.

Cannabis can be a great tool for those who suffer from MS by providing relief and helping to control symptoms of pain, stiffness, muscle spasms and helping to battle depression.

There is additional evidence that has been reported in which specific cannabinoids have been able to help those suffering from MS in regards to sleep issues, fibromyalgia and other medical conditions as well.

Currently, there are two forms of synthetic marijuana that have been FDA approved specifically for MS patients which are taken in capsule form, orally.

With that said, most experts agree in the thinking that the real benefits and relief should be experienced through the actual cannabis plant in its natural form.

MS sufferers can especially benefit from high CBD strains or ratio (CBD:THC) products to help with pain, fatigue and depression.

Numerous studies have been done and research seems to point to the fact that cannabinoids have a favorable impact in helping MS patients with various forms of pain and spasticity.

Insomnia

According to SleepAdvisor.org, <u>30% of the adult U.S. population suffers from insomnia and 10% suffer from chronic insomnia.</u>

Insomnia can be described as having difficulty falling asleep or staying asleep, even when a person has the opportunity to and/or despite the fact the person may be exhausted.

People who suffer from insomnia often have accompanying symptoms such as fatigue, low energy, inability to focus, mood disturbances and overall decreased performance.

Additionally, insomnia is thought to be linked to other medical or psychiatric issues although we cannot yet sufficiently correlate to what extent.

Insomnia is characterized by two different types:

- *Acute Insomnia*
- *Chronic Insomnia*

Acute insomnia is typically brief and it's directly related to emotions and current life circumstances or events such as worrying about an upcoming deadline or project, hearing devastating news, etc.

In most circumstances, people with acute insomnia find the problem tends to take care of itself without any treatment needed.

Chronic insomnia is characterized by disrupted sleep that occurs for at least three or more nights per week, lasting at least three months.

There are a multitude of different things that can cause insomnia such as poor sleep habits, changes of environment, medications, work schedules/hours worked, clinical disorders and more.

Over time, these consistent patterns of insufficient sleep become your normal routine and your body adapts despite the much-needed sleep.

Current treatment of Insomnia:
There are many basic, common sense-based tactics that people can deploy such as:

- Maintaining a regular sleep schedule
- Avoiding caffeine and other stimulants before bed
- Avoiding bright screens and lights before bed
- Avoiding eating before bed
- Regular exercise
- Meditation and other relaxing techniques

If these natural measures don't work, some patients turn to over the counter sleeping aids and antihistamines to induce drowsiness.

In more serious cases, patients seek out a doctor who may prescribe sleeping pills or other forms of treatment.

How Cannabis Can Help

Cannabis could be the perfect solution for many people who suffer with trouble sleeping.

It's an especially perfect solution for those who would prefer a more natural form of treatment as opposed to opting for over the counter or prescription drugs.

Cannabis Indica would be the ideal choice as it focuses its effect more on the body and is typically associated with feelings of sedation and relaxation.

There are various different Indica strains and each strain can have different effects unique to each person. In addition to strains effecting individuals uniquely, the amount you consume will also have a direct effect on your experience which means that patients will have to experiment with different strains and titrating dosages before finding out what works best for them individually.

Interestingly enough, older cannabis that is exposed to oxygen over long periods of time, begins to undergo a process where some of the THC changes to CBN or cannabinol.

The cannabis' Phyto cannabinoids that undergo this transformation are shown to be up to five times more sedating than the original compound! But, with that being said, CBN can take years to form and it's extremely hard to find strains of cannabis with high amounts of CBN.

In regards to the topic of Cannabis and sleep, an article on TheSleepDoctor.com references a study on Cannabis and Insomnia, by Rolando Tringale, MD and Claudia Jensen, MD.

This study concluded the following:
"Patients seeking physician approval to use cannabis commonly report benefits on decreasing sleep latency, even if a sleep disorder is not the chief complaint. This previously unreported result is supported by recent findings concerning the endocannabinoid system, as well as voluminous anecdotal evidence. Larger double-blinded studies are indicated to rigorously explore this important clinical effect."

This research showed us that patients typically reported that cannabis helped them to fall asleep quicker, regardless of whether or not the patient suffered from insomnia.

There are various different ways to consume cannabis with a variety of different onset times.

For Sleep: *(Indica Strains Are Recommended)*

Smoking/Inhalation: It has a quick onset (within minutes) and you can choose to do it within the hour or two before you go to bed in order to help relax/sedate you. This can be done both through smoking the actual plant or through the use of vaporizing devices and THC derived oils.

There is a lot in the news now about the safety of vaporizing and the linking of vaporizers to teen deaths and popcorn lung. It's too early to put any definitive labels on the safety of vaping, but it's important that people understand what it is exactly that they are vaping.

For instance, many of these vaping issues may be arising due to clandestine dealers cutting the THC oil with fillers such as propylene glycol. According to the Agency For Toxic Substances & Disease Registry, propylene glycol is "used by the chemical, food, and pharmaceutical industries as an antifreeze when leakage might lead to contact with food."

In regards to vaping, a reputable medical cannabis dispensary will have products with either straight THC concentrate oils that have no cutting agent OR if there is a cutting agent used, it would be something natural like MCT oil or coconut oil.

Sublingual: You can use an oral syringe or tincture and disperse the substance under your tongue where it is absorbed into your bloodstream by dissolving through the tissue in your mouth (under your tongue, gums and cheeks). Because this is going directly to your bloodstream, it's a fairly quick onset time.

Orally: In this instance, you would most likely be looking at oral capsules, RSO, tinctures or edibles. The typically onset time is about two hours (although this can range on an individual level due to unique biochemistry, metabolism, etc.).

Post-Traumatic Stress Disorder (PTSD)

Post-Traumatic Stress Disorder, which is most commonly referred to as "PTSD," is a mental health condition that can affect anyone who's experienced or witnessed a terrifying, life-threatening or traumatic experience.

We often associate this disease with soldiers that have gone to war and come back, but it also affects a great number of other people who've suffered through natural disasters, serious accidents, terrorist attacks, sexual assaults, etc.

Those who suffer with PTSD often have symptoms that include flashbacks, nightmares and forms of severe anxiety such as uncontrollable thoughts about the experience.

Additionally, many people with this disorder will avoid particular people, places and things that they associate with the experience or particular memories.

Common Symptoms of Those Who Suffer With PTSD:
- Depression
- Memory issues
- Changes in personality

- Substance abuse

According to the U.S. Department of Veteran Affairs :

The following statistics are based on the U.S. population

- *7-8% of people will have PTSD at some point in their lives*
- *About 8 million adults suffer from PTSD each year*
- *10% of Women will develop PTSD in their lives*
- *4% of Men will develop PTSD in their lives*

Current treatment of PTSD:

At the moment, it's sad to say that most PTSD treatment consists mainly of therapy and antidepressants or sleeping pills.

With the therapy approach, the ideal goal is to improve the patient's symptoms and help them to develop the skills they need to deal with their trauma and to restore a sense of confidence or some sort of positive shift in their lives.

Two common types of PTSD Therapy include:

Cognitive Processing Therapy:

Speaking with your therapist about the event and how it affects your thoughts, your life and your outlook. Often referred to as CPT, Cognitive Processing Therapy looks to examine how patients think about their trauma and help them to discover ways of living with it.

Prolonged Exposure Therapy:

This type of approach focuses on helping patients to confront memories or things that they associate with the traumatic event. Typically, it includes anywhere from eight to fifteen sessions with a duration of an hour and half per session.

This can include teaching different breathing techniques, meditations, the practice of recounting traumatic memories and experiences, listening to recordings of yourself to reflect/confront these feelings and a variety of other thoughtful tactics to help patients ease their symptoms.

Eye Movement Desensitization and Reprocessing (EMDR):

As opposed to telling your therapist about your experiences, with EMDR your focus is instead being shifted to concentrating on your therapist as you watch and listen to them. This may include using hand movements, making sounds, flashing lights etc. with the goal of being able to get the patient to associate some form of positivity with these traumatic experiences they are being asked to recall. This can take a couple months of consistent weekly sessions before seeing any progress.

Medication:

As a last resort, those who will do anything to get relief will seek out medications such as antipsychotic prescription drugs, anti-depressants, beta blockers, benzodiazepines, and monoamine oxidase inhibitors.

Common PTSD medications prescribed for anxiety include:

- *Prozac*
- *Paxil*
- *Zoloft*
- *Effexor*

How Cannabis Can Help

It's important to preface this with the fact that regular therapy is typically recommended in conjunction with cannabis treatment in order to achieve maximum results. This combination shows great promise in regards to providing relief to those who suffer from Post-Traumatic Stress Disorder.

People who suffer from PTSD have been found to have an endocannabinoid deficiency, which makes cannabis a perfect treatment due its ability to work naturally with the human endocannabinoid system.

Cannabis contains different cannabinoids, such as the ones we've mentioned in previous sections of this book, which can play key roles in assisting PTSD patients who are deficient in these cannabinoids.

Cannabis has been reported to help prevent the retrieval of underlying trauma, reduce/prevent memories and nightmares and can even help patients to attain an increased sense of well-being.

It does this by helping to fill missing gaps in the endocannabinoid system of these PTSD patients, who have a deficiency in which they are lacking many of these cannabinoids.

According to an article on <u>**HealthCareInAmerica.US**</u>:

"A study conducted by NYU Langone Medical Center researchers showed that people suffering from PTSD have much lower levels of a neurotransmitter called anandamide than others. Anandamide is one of the body's primary endocannabinoids, meaning natural cannabinoids produced by the body. These operate in a similar way to cannabis by stimulating the endocannabinoid system, which is responsible for core functions such as mood, happiness, fear, and anxiety."

In that same HealthCareInAmerica.US article, Dr. Alexander Neumeister stated:

"There's a consensus among clinicians that existing pharmaceutical treatments such as antidepressant simply do not work. In fact, we know very well that people with PTSD who use marijuana — a potent cannabinoid — often experience more relief from their symptoms than they do from

antidepressants and other psychiatric medications. Clearly, there's a very urgent need to develop novel evidence-based treatments for PTSD."

– Dr. Alexander Neumeister

Additionally, CBD has been shown to assist in disrupting the frequency of long-term traumatic memory, helping it to hopefully, eventually slowly fade away.

In contrast to prescription medications, cannabis allows patients to still maintain some sense of clear headed-ness and awareness as opposed to feelings of "numbness," which can sometimes be the way patients have described the feelings of being on prescription drugs such as opioids.

Due to the fact that high THC strains can aggravate anxiety in some PTSD patients, it's recommended that PTSD patients look for a high CBD strain or Ratio (CBD:THC:$\Delta8$) product to start.

Eventually, patients will slowly build up a tolerance to THC, but if they decide to go that route, it's important to start low and go slow with dosages until you know how it affects you uniquely.

Although cannabis alone is not the solution, it seems as though it's become a safer and healthier way for patients to process trauma in a manner that may be more suitable and effective. This, in combination to therapy, provides patients the best overall results in regards to developing skills to deal with trauma and helping to promote a positive shift in their lives.

Nausea

Everyone has experienced nausea at some point or another. For those who need a refresher, nausea is when you begin feeling sick in your stomach, your repulsed by the idea of any type of food, and it's accompanied by a constant feeling of needing to vomit.

Although nausea is something we've all experienced at some point or another, it can be the result of different circumstances in each case.

For instance, nausea can occur the morning after a long night of drinking with friends, while at the same time, someone else may be experiencing nausea due to side effects from medications; such as those from cancer patients looking to curb feelings of nausea from their chemotherapy treatment.

In fact, many patients who've undergone chemotherapy don't respond well to treatments using traditional drugs, which can actually make them feel more lethargic, "zoned out" and sometimes delusional.

Generally, nausea can be induced by:

- Motion sickness
- Food Poisoning

- Pregnancy
- Flu symptoms
- Infections
- Side effects from treatments *(Example)* – Chemotherapy
- Among others

For the most part, nausea is short lived and it's something that comes and goes in a manner that most people can suffer through. But, there are some cases in which people can have forms of chronic nausea, in which they battle with every day. This can be due to a variety of reasons and/or health concerns, as well as outside factors like stress and anxiety.

Current (Non-Cannabis) Forms of Treating Nausea:

There are plenty of medications that can be used to get rid of nausea, especially when it becomes persistent. With that being said, these over the counter medications and prescriptions can come with unwanted side effects such as diarrhea, constipation, sleeping issues, headaches and more.

How Cannabis Can Help

For the most part, those who are familiar with cannabis are well aware of its amazing ability to help with nausea and headaches.

Familiarity aside, we now have actual evidence through multiple clinical trials such as those from PubMed, that have come to the same conclusion.

Cannabis is not only a great way to help alleviate nausea, but it can actually be a great way to help battle some of the negative side effects of nausea by helping to stimulate appetite, increase energy, elevate mood and help those suffering to feel better overall.

We even have evidence regarding studies dating back to the 1970's which have well documented the effectiveness that cannabis has had in treating the many unpleasant and sometimes unbearable feelings of nausea.

Cannabis is a great choice for battling nausea because it's literally treating your symptoms at the source by interacting naturally with our endocannabinoid system.

Nausea is a sensation that is typically created and regulated by our bodies central nervous system and endocannabinoid system. Our bodies send neurotransmitters to communicate within these systems in order to help regulate everything from our mood, fertility, sleep, memory and even pain sensation.

For those of you that may be older in age, yet new to the modern world of cannabis, or perhaps those who are hesitant to get "high" ... there is some promise in regards to CBD's effects with nausea as well.

According to an article on Eaze.com and the British Journal of Pharmacology:

"A 2012 study showed promise for the anti-emetic (nausea- and vomiting-fighting) properties of CBD, the second-most common cannabinoid–and one that doesn't get you high. In it, Canadian and Israeli researchers found that CBD produced strong anti-emetic/anti-nausea effects in rats by interacting with the body's abundant 5-HT1A autoreceptors. More research is needed to determine whether CBD alone is an effective anti-emetic in humans. And conventional wisdom has it that THC and CBD are both better when working as a team; that thinking drives the popularity of tinctures and vaporizers with CBD-to-THC ratios like 3:1 and vice versa."

For those who have been paying attention up to this point of this book, you'll notice that the information listed above, references 'THC and CBD ...better working as a team...," which you might recall is something referred to as the "Entourage Effect," discussed in earlier chapters in this book.

Anxiety and Depression

Anxiety and Depression are being grouped together because unfortunately, a great number of those whose suffer with one, also suffer with the other. Additionally, both anxiety and depression have causes, symptoms and treatments that often times overlap.

In fact, *according* to the Anxiety and Depression Association of America:

"Nearly one-half of those diagnosed with depression are also diagnosed with an anxiety disorder."

And according to HealthLine.com, an estimated *16.2 million adults living in the United States (6.7%), have experienced at the very least, one major depressive episode within a given year.*

These serious, yet common mental disorders have the ability to affect our feelings, thoughts, motivation, mood, sleep and social life just to name a few.

Symptoms Can Include:

- Depressed mood
- Lack of energy
- Increased OR Decreased appetite
- Lack of confidence and feelings of worthlessness

- Irritability
- Anxiousness or hyper anxiousness
- Insomnia
- Feelings of guilt
- Trouble concentrating
- Having suicidal thoughts or behaviors

Current treatments of Anxiety & Depression:
At the moment, the two most popular forms of treating depression are:
Psychotherapy *(A.K.A. – "Talk Therapy")* – This is aimed at helping people to identify and change unwanted thoughts, emotions and behaviors by scheduling appointments with a licensed mental healthcare professional.

Medications – Antidepressants are the form of medication prescribed for people suffering from depression. Common examples of antidepressants include Zoloft, Prozac and Lexapro.

Other forms of dealing with depression might include:

- Exercise
- Meditation
- Support groups
- Adopting a pet
- Immersing yourself in a new hobby or interest

How Cannabis Can Help

As we know from earlier chapters, cannabis works with our body's endocannabinoid system and helps our body to maintain homeostasis *along with guiding our mood* and overall health.

Additionally, cannabis is known for its amazing ability to help ease feelings of stress and anxiety, which are two feelings that are strongly associated with depression.

With that being said, it's extremely important to consider titration (dosing) methods that lean more conservative. This is because consuming too much can sometimes produce the opposite effect your looking for, which could result in paranoia or feelings of discomfort or even anxiety.

On the other hand, by taking just the right amount or even micro dosing throughout the day, patients have been able to find a great deal of hope and relief. A micro dose would typically be anything under 10mg, depending on the individual and their tolerance.

Regardless of cannabis and depression being a fairly new area of study, anytime you're talking about mental health it can become extremely complex as there are so many different factors at play.

For instance, when assessing the effects of cannabis use in regards to anxiety and depression, there is a deeper associated context that is variable within each person along with other factors such as current circumstances, temperament, family history, etc... This might help to explain why past research surrounding this issue has shown unpredictable and inconclusive results.

According to a study by the National Center for Biotechnology information:

*** Note: "HA" stands for "Harm Avoidance" which is something associated with those suffering from depression and is characterized by heightened feelings of apprehension, shyness & pessimism. ***

"While HA likely increases anxiety and depression, marijuana can have anxiolytic (anti-anxiety) and euphoriant effects. Such positive mood effects are reported among the top motives for marijuana use (Lee et al., 2009; Newcomb et al., 1998; Simons et al., 1998). Marijuana use may also facilitate social contact (Green & Ritter, 2000) which could, in turn, improve mood and ultimately mental health. Animal research suggests a direct anxiolytic effect of cannabis administration (e.g., Guimaraes et al., 1990; Soares et al., 2010; for a review, see Mechoulam, Parker, & Gallily, 2002). The exact mechanism of these effects has not been *determined, although they seem to be restricted to the effects of cannabidiol and not Δ9-tetrahydrocannabinol (e.g., Zuardi et al., 2006) and likely involve serotonergic receptors in the dorsal periaqueductal gray matter as the basis for anxiolytic effects (Soares et al., 2010). The potential for marijuana use to affect mood suggests a possible moderating role of marijuana on the relation of HA to anxiety and depression. Specifically, to the degree that marijuana produces anxiolytic and/or euphoriant effects – either directly through its biochemical effects on neurotransmitters and receptors or indirectly through expectations and/or the facilitation of mood and beneficial social interactions – marijuana use may buffer individuals high in HA from increased risk for anxiety and depression."*

Current studies, such as the one above, are considered anecdotal evidence as there is still much research that needs to be done and clinical trials to be had. It's also extremely important to remember that mental health is a complex area of study with various contributing factors at play. With that being said, things look hopeful and promising for cannabis when it comes to helping to treat depression and anxiety.

Glaucoma

Glaucoma is a condition in which your eye's optic nerve is damaged due to a buildup of fluid and pressure, usually occurring in the front part of your eye. The disease can affect anyone and it accounts for approximately 10% percent of all blindness in the U.S., while remaining the second-leading cause of blindness worldwide.

The increased "intraocular pressure" in glaucoma patients, damages the optic nerve in the eye which in turn transmits images to the brain which can sometimes appear as "rainbow colored rings" or "halos around lights." Continued damage to the optic nerve can result in a permanent loss of vision and if left untreated, those affected will become blind within just a few years.

It's usually recommended to get your vision checked at least once a year as most people who suffer from glaucoma have no early symptoms.

Although the cause of glaucoma is largely unclear, it's believed that factors such genetics, ethnicity, health problems such as diabetes, and family history play a role. Additionally, the risk of glaucoma increases with age despite the fact it has the ability to affect anyone from children to the elderly.

Current treatment of Glaucoma:
There are various forms of treatments used to help glaucoma patients reduce the buildup of fluid in their eye, thus decreasing intraocular pressure.

Some current forms of Glaucoma treatment include:

- *Prescription eye drops*
- *Prescription medication (which helps to curb fluid buildup)*
- *Laser surgery*
- *Micro surgery (trabeculectomy – surgery in which the doctor builds a new channel for draining the fluid to help ease eye pressure)*

Unfortunately, there is no cure for glaucoma and some of the above treatments can cause side effects such as allergies to medications, irritation, stinging, redness, blurred vision and in some cases, can even cause retinal detachment.

But, perhaps there may be another way…

How Cannabis Can Help

The neuroprotective properties of cannabis can potentially help play a role by inhibiting the advancement of glaucoma in those who suffer.

Additionally, cannabis has shown to be very effective in treating intraocular pressure, the only drawback being that the effects only last for a couple hours.

This means the patient must consistently consume cannabis throughout the day in order to solely treat the condition with cannabis alone. With that being said, cannabis can be extremely effective when used in combination with traditional glaucoma treatments.

Doctors and scientists are looking at developing a new form of glaucoma specific treatment through THC eye drops, which would give patients the ability to distribute the medicine directly to the eye. Due to this route of administration direct to the source, patients wouldn't have to deal with the psychoactive effects typically associated with THC.

According to a 1971 study, which looked at the ability and effects of smoking cannabis in glaucoma patients, cannabis showed the ability to decrease intraocular pressure by 25%.

Often times glaucoma patients suffer severe headaches as well, which are usually due to optic nerve pain and it's extremely common in the latter stages of glaucoma.

The analgesic and anti-inflammatory effects associated with the consumption of cannabis allow it to act as a powerful pain reliever and it can help to reduce the swelling of the optic nerve.

Nausea and vomiting are other symptoms that have been associated with glaucoma patients and as we know from prior chapters, cannabis works great in helping patients to relive such symptoms.

PMS

Premenstrual syndrome, better known as *"PMS,"* refers to the multiple different symptoms that women suffer from prior to getting their period. This is caused by hormone fluctuations that arise after a woman ovulates.

Typically, PMS symptoms occur about a week or so before women get their period and they can present themselves through physical, emotional or behavioral forms.

Physical Symptoms Can Include:

- Feeling bloated
- Nausea
- Cramping
- Tenderness in breasts
- Weight gain
- Constipation or diarrhea
- Headaches

Emotional Symptoms Can Include:

- Feeling tense or anxious
- Mood swings
- Feelings of depression
- Crying outbursts
- Not being able to sleep
- Irritability

Behavioral Symptoms Can Include:

- Forgetfulness
- Difficulty focusing/concentrating
- Lack of energy

PMS can also affect other conditions, worsening symptoms for women who also suffer from conditions such chronic fatigue, anxiety and irritable bowel syndrome (IBS) to name a few.

Simple ways to help mitigate PMS symptoms:

- *Going to the gym or doing yoga*
- *Meditation*
- *Getting a good night sleep (at least 8 hours)*
- *Not smoking cigarettes/tobacco*
- *Avoiding too much caffeine*
- *Maintaining a healthy diet*

Other options can include medication such as over-the-counter pain medication, antianxiety medication, antidepressants or birth control pills. Other supplements that may be recommended include vitamin B, vitamin D and making sure to get enough calcium.

For some women, symptoms are worse than they are for others.

How Cannabis Can Help

Just as with many of the other conditions in this book, cannabis can be an amazing tool to help battle these symptoms in addition to some of the traditional methods listed above.

As we've already learned up to this point, cannabis is able to help treat such a long list of ailments due to the fact that we have cannabinoid receptors all throughout our body.

Cannabis has had many well documented affects when it comes to a myriad of conditions, including many symptoms associated with PMS such as:

- *Pain relief/decreased breast tenderness*
- *Helping to treat and ease the pain of headaches*
- *Calming gastrointestinal issues*
- *Aiding in sleep*
- *Helping to stabilize mood and battle depression*

There are many ways in which cannabis alone would be a great option for women suffering through the symptoms of PMS. Typically, most women will get optimal results in using cannabis in addition to any traditional methods that they may already be successfully using to treat such symptoms.

Arthritis

Arthritis is a joint disease or joint pain and it's made up of a variety of over a hundred different types of conditions. Arthritis does not discriminate and can affect people of all ages, sexes and races.

In fact, according to the Arthritis Foundation, arthritis is said to be the leading cause of disability in America and it affects over 50 Million adults and 300,000 children.

Common Symptoms of Arthritis include:

- Swelling
- Pain
- Stiffness
- Decreased range of motion

These symptoms can vary in each case and sometimes symptoms even come and go, ranging from mild or moderate to severe.

Arthritis is something that may get worse over time, which can result in chronic pain and make it difficult to accomplish daily activities. In some cases, arthritis can actually cause permanent changes in your joint(s) and there are even some forms of arthritis that can affect other areas of your body such as the heart, eyes, lungs, kidneys and skin in addition to your joints.

Common types of Arthritis include:
Osteoarthritis:
This is the most common type of arthritis and it causes the cartilage between our bones to wear away, resulting in bone rubbing on bone which leads to pain, swelling and stiffness.

Osteoarthritis is typically managed with hot/cold application, muscle and joint exercises and over the counter medication.

Inflammatory Arthritis:
Inflammatory arthritis is a condition in which your immune system goes awry and it begins attacking your joints, internal organs, eyes and other parts of your body.

Rheumatoid arthritis and *psoriatic arthritis* are each examples of different forms of inflammatory arthritis. These forms of arthritis are currently being treated with disease modifying antirheumatic drugs or *"DMARDs."*

The best-case scenario is to catch the arthritis early with the goal being to achieve remission in order to prevent any permanent joint damage.

Other forms of arthritis can occur through infectious bacteria, viruses, diseases or fungus that can cause joint inflammation. In some cases, there is a buildup of uric acid in the body which can result in Gout.

Over the Counter Treatment of Arthritis:
Current over the counter treatments of arthritis can include analgesics such as Tylenol, Percocet and Vicodin which are prescribed to help ease the pain.

Other forms of treatments can include topical creams which contain menthol, capsaicin or Advil. Additionally, Motrin or Aleve can be used to help reduce pain and inflammation.

How Cannabis Can Help

Those who suffer with arthritis often contain unusually high amounts of CB2 receptors in their affected joints, which makes cannabis an excellent option for treatment.

Researcher Jason McDougall reports that cannabinoids such as THC and CBD, control the firing of pain signals from our joints to our brain by sticking themselves to nerve receptors.

This news shows great promise to those who suffer from arthritis and according to an article on the Canadian Arthritis Society's website, Arthritis.ca; *"An estimated two thirds of Canadians who use cannabis for medical purposes do so to help manage arthritis symptoms."*

CBD may help alleviate arthritis associated symptoms such as pain, insomnia, and anxiety. As always, it's important to start with low dosages and to buy from a reputable company that tests each batch for purity and potency. Most reputable companies get 3rd party lab results in conjunction to their own testing which guarantees purity and transparency.

This new trend of growing popularity centered around CBD is coming at a time where CBD is becoming more readily available.

Industry reports are showing that people who suffer from arthritis are among the top buyers of CBD products with their leading reason for purchase being pain relief.

There have also been reports showing that THC has been found to be a much more powerful solution in treating inflammation when being compared to hydrocortisone and it has twenty times the power of Asprin!

CBD is also a great solution to finding anti-inflammatory relief. CBD and THC topical creams can be applied directly to the source of pain to provide more targeted forms of relief.

Other routes of treatment can include tinctures, vaporizers or smoking the cannabis flower.

Not only is cannabis an amazing source of pain relief for those who suffer from arthritis, but it's equally as effective in treating inflammation symptoms as well.

The combination of CBD and THC in helping to treat and battle symptoms of arthritis are a perfect example of how different cannabinoids can work together to provide even stronger results.

Migraines

Migraines are intense and severe headaches that are usually accompanied by additional symptoms such as:

- Nausea
- Pain behind the ears, eyes or temples
- Seeing spots or lights
- Being sensitive to both light and sound
- Vomiting
- In some cases, temporary vision loss

Migraines are more extreme than normal headaches, which are characterized by an unpleasant pain in your head usually targeting the forehead, temples, or back of your neck. Typically, these are tension headaches that are caused by stress, muscle strain, anxiety and sometimes fatigue.

Migraines can be debilitating and really affect the quality of life for those who suffer from them. This makes finding relief a top priority and it's important to consider how you decide to treat your migraine.

Current treatment of Migraines:
Migraines are being treated with various over the counter medications such as aspirin and ibuprofen.

But, often times these over the counter remedies don't work and people need something stronger.

Prescription drugs such as codeine or oxycodone, which are both opioids, are prescribed to patients and we've learned in early chapters how dangerous, harmful and addictive these opioids can become.

Fortunately, many are finding out there is a more natural way to treat migraines and find relief from the pain and other additional symptoms associated with migraines.

How Cannabis Can Help

Cannabis is an extremely powerful solution in battling migraines as it has the ability to essentially attack the migraine from a variety of different fronts by helping to simultaneously treat pain, nausea and inflammation.

According to WebMD.Com, there was a study done at the University of Colorado in which 121 people who suffered from regular migraines, used cannabis daily to prevent migraine attacks.

The results yielded that an incredible 40% of those who participated said the number of migraines they typically get were cut in half!

The participants used a variety of different strains of cannabis and mostly chose to inhale as it was a quicker onset method and helped to ease migraine pain faster. Edible products were also used, but the edibles did not seem to be as effective.

There is not much research to lean on as studies have been either limited or non-existent due to the Schedule I restrictions around Cannabis, but there has been much success in anecdotal testing that warrants claims for clinical trials.

An article on Migraine.Com describes a presentation that was given to the Congress of the European Academy of Neurology in 2017. Italian researchers brought forth evidence supporting the use of cannabis for both preventing and treating acute migraines.

These researchers first set out to study how to properly dose cannabis for usage.

In the study, a group of 48 people who suffered from chronic migraines were administered medical cannabis with varying levels of THC and CBD through oral doses.

Results found that typically, with an oral dose of 200mg, acute pain was relieved by up to 55%.

The second phase of the research included 79 people who suffer from chronic migraines and they received either a dose of cannabis *OR* amitriptyline which is a common antidepressant used to treat migraines.

Participants were able to use 200mg of cannabis for any acute attacks that occurred.

In a three-month period, the people who were administered the cannabis had a roughly 40.4% reduction in migraine attacks.

Additionally, researchers were able to find that cannabis was extremely effective in treating acute pain from migraines by reducing pain intensity by up to 43.5%.

The most common side effects that were associated with cannabis treatment included drowsiness and a difficulty in concentrating. Some participants even mentioned an improvement in stomach aches and musculoskeletal pain.

There is still much research to be done on cannabis and its effects on treating migraines. Although we still need to see clinical trials start taking place, for now cannabis holds a lot of promise in helping to treat migraines and there is a growing amount of anecdotal evidence supporting such claims.

Anorexia

According to the National Association of Anorexia Nervosa and Associated Disorders, there are roughly 8 million people in the U.S. (approximately 3% of the population) who suffer from anorexia nervosa, bulimia or other related eating disorders.

This life-threatening eating disorder and metabolic condition also has psychological and emotional tendencies which usually results in excessive weight loss and extreme thinness, due to starvation.

Although, it is possible to be normal weight or sometimes even overweight and still be affected by this disorder.

Those who suffer from anorexia are consumed by their own efforts to control their body shape and size.

So what causes anorexia?
The root cause of anorexia is usually psychological, but it can be attributed to several other sociocultural factors, genetics, obsessive compulsive personality traits and other neurobiological factors.

Anorexia Signs & Symptoms:

- Lying about eating habits
- Irritability
- Skewed perception of body weight
- Obsessive thoughts and behavior pertaining to weight gain
- Feeling insecure
- Decreased interest in sex
- Anxiety and depression
- Suicidal thoughts

Anorexia has a frightening mortality rate and the highest of any other mental illness.

Current treatment of Anorexia:

After someone has been diagnosed with Anorexia, they will typically undergo a variety of treatment including psychotherapy, medical treatment and nutrition counseling.

Mental health professionals who treat anorexia may draw from a variety of different styles of therapy when treating patients and trying to help them in their recovery.

Cognitive behavioral therapy is typically used in order to create a safe "talk therapy" environment in which patients can begin understanding how their negative thoughts and feelings about themselves and their image are connected to their disorder.

This also can help patients to learn and recognize positive and negative patterns that may lead to success or relapse.

In terms of medical treatment, there are typically no drugs that are prescribed for the disease itself, but more for symptoms that go along with it such as depression and anxiety for example.

Other forms of non-prescription treatment could be recommended as well such as meditation, yoga, spin class, etc. These are prescribed mostly to help elevate mood, build body image and lower stress levels.

Nutritionists are also provided to help those who suffer to better understand good eating habits and how to achieve a healthy, well-balanced diet. This allows the person to understand not only what they should be consuming, but how much and why.

How Cannabis Can Help

As we know at this point, our endocannabinoid system plays a big role in our body maintaining homeostasis. This is extremely interesting as it pertains to eating disorders because they cause imbalances in our body's homeostasis.

This leads to suggestions that perhaps cannabis and many of its cannabinoids could help to treat patients suffering from a variety of eating disorders.

Two examples that may easily demonstrate this point can be provided by looking at two different cannabinoids in THC and THCV.

Often times THC can be known to stimulate appetite and cause what most people refer to as "the munchies." THCV on the other hand, is a cannabinoid that actually helps to suppress appetite as it's an antagonist of CB1 and CB2 receptors by blocking THC.

Cannabis has also been known to increase people's senses, including people's sense of smell and taste. This can help those who suffer to start finding joy in the pleasure of eating, which could be exceptionally beneficial to someone who is only used to associating negative thoughts and thinking patterns with eating.

In the case of anorexia, we'd be looking at the appetite stimulating effects that THC causes.

Patients may find relief from other symptoms by consuming cannabis as well such as depression, stress, and anxiety. By choosing a strain that induces positive and energetic effects, like a Sativa or Sativa dominant Hybrid.

Some strains can help patients to deal with feelings of self-consciousness and allow them to feel less worried or pressured when it comes to counting calories. Remember, each strain can affect everyone differently, thus people may experience different effects with the same strain and it's important to find out what works best for you and your body.

In one study done in Denmark, which was done with anorexic patients, those who received a synthetic form of THC gained more weight than the subjects who were given the placebo.

Additionally, there has been substantial research and clinical studies done that have proven the effectiveness of cannabis as an appetite stimulant for people suffering from cancer and HIV/AIDS.

With that said, there has been very little research in specifically how cannabis can be used to help treat anorexia. Things look very promising, but there needs to be more clinical trials and research done specifically looking into how it helps to treat those who suffer with anorexia.

Cannabis is certainly something that is providing much hope and it seems to be effective in helping to treat a variety of unwanted symptoms associated with anorexia and other eating disorders.

Cancer

According to Healthline.com, cancer is the second leading cause of death in the United States behind heart disease and both have been the top 2 leading causes of death for more than a decade in America.

Cancer is a disease that occurs when there is an uncontrolled growth of abnormal cells in the body which crowd out the normal cells, making it hard for the body to perform and work the way it's supposed to.

The accumulation of these extra cells may form a giant mass of tissue, called a tumor. Tumors can either be benign (non-cancerous) or malignant (cancerous).

Some current forms of cancer treatment include:
- *Surgery*
- *Chemotherapy*
- *Radiation*
- *A combination of both radiation and chemotherapy treatment*

Surgery may be performed to remove cancerous tumors in which the doctor may remove all or some of the body parts affected by the cancer. Surgery is not always an option for all forms of cancer, as some such as leukemia are best treated with drugs and often times, cancer requires chemotherapy or radiation treatment.

Chemotherapy can be given through an IV and also in the form of pills that are taken orally. This drug is used to kill cancer cells and to stop these cells from growing and multiplying. Chemo drugs travel through the entire body which make them beneficial for targeting cancer that quickly spreads throughout the body.

There are some extremely terrible side effects in using chemotherapy despite its effectiveness in killing cancer cells. Chemo also kills healthy cells in the body as well, which is the reason for many of the terrible side effects associated with the drug.

Some of these side effects include *extreme fatigue, depression, loss of appetite, hair loss, nausea and vomiting* just to name a few.

Radiation, which can cause many of the same negative side effects of chemotherapy, is used to target cancer cells by using high doses of radiation. It's often times used in combination with surgery or chemotherapy and it's similar to getting an x-ray.

Common side effects Associated with current cancer treatments:

- Loss of appetite
- Hair loss
- Problems sleeping and extreme fatigue
- Diarrhea
- Fertility issues
- Edema
- Anemia

How Cannabis Can Help

Cannabis is a perfect fit when it comes to helping to treat cancer symptoms.

In fact, cannabis helps to treat a majority of the symptoms that affect cancer patients such as:

- Nausea
- Anxiety
- Pain
- Helps treat inflammation
- Helps to stimulate appetite
- Headaches
- Gastrointestinal problems
- Mood

Additionally, Delta 8, Delta 9 and CBD were ALL shown to possess the ability to stop the growth of tumors as we've learned in the earlier chapters of this book.

One such example of a form of medicinal cannabis that has shown to be particularly effective in battling cancer is something known as "Rick Simpson Oil."

Rick Simpson Oil or RSO, is a highly concentrated form of pure cannabis oil.

In 1997, Rick Simpson was an engineer working in a Canadian hospital boiler room where he was covering asbestos with aerosol glue on the hospital's pipes. He inhaled toxic and poisonous fumes which caused his nervous system to go into a temporary shock in which he passed out and woke up in the emergency room.

After his accident, he suffered from a constant ringing in his ear and dizzy spells. It seemed as though all of the medications the doctor gave him were ineffective and often times instead made symptoms worse.

After seeing a documentary on the benefits of cannabis and its positive medicinal effects, Rick went to his doctor.

His doctor refused to even consider using cannabis for treatment, so Rick then took matters into his own hands and found a way to get the cannabis himself. After beginning using cannabis, Rick began to see significant improvement in his tinnitus and some of his other symptoms that he had suffered from his incident.

Later, in 2003, Rick began to see various suspicious bumps that appeared on his arm. After having a biopsy performed, the doctor confirmed that

Rick had basal cell carcinoma, a form of skin cancer.

After successfully treating his previous ailments with cannabis, Rick read about a study done by the Journal of the National Cancer Institute in which cannabis had been used to kill cancer cells in mice.

So, Rick did some research and created his own highly concentrated form of cannabis oil, in which he applied directly to his skin and covered the affected area with a bandage for several days.

After just 4 days, Rick removed the bandages and the cancerous growths were nowhere to be found.

To learn more about Rick Simpson Oil and even how to make your own, you can search Google or if you have the eBook, you can check out this article link from Leafly.

Rick Simpson Oil is not the only cannabis product that helps to fight cancer.

An article by the National Cancer Institute titled *"Cannabis and Cannabinoids (PDQ®)–Health Professional Version,"* on cancer.gov, outlines a brief summary regarding their overview of the subject matter.

Some of the things they discuss include how cannabis has been used for thousands of years for medicinal purposes and how cannabinoids may be beneficial in treating cancer-related side effects and symptoms.

In fact, cannabis has been so effective in the treating of cancer related symptoms, that in some cases patients are often able to stop using a variety of other medications that they were prescribed, which eliminated all the associated side effects related to their prescriptions.

Furthermore, cannabis is a FAR more attractive route of treatment in that it's a natural form of medication and its side effects are not remotely dangerous. Contrary to the side effects of many other medications, associated side effects of cannabis are often instead sought out after, as these effects tend to coincidentally be forms of treatment.

(Ex.) – THC may cause the munchies, which might be something sought out after by someone suffering from cancer or anorexia.

To sum it up, cannabis and a variety of its cannabinoids in particular, have shown to not only fight and prevent the growth of cancer cells, but also to help treat a variety of symptoms related to current treatments involving the use of chemotherapy and radiation.

Delta 8 is especially interesting when dealing specifically with nausea and appetite, showing to be

100% more effective than Delta 9. On the flip side, Delta 9 is more effective in treating pain symptoms.

In today's modern world of medicinal cannabis, there are products such as vape cartridges that contain ratio amounts of cannabinoids, such as CBD, Delta 8 and Delta 9 which work together to treat a variety of different symptoms and give patients maximum forms of relief. These may work particularly well with cancer patients.

Conclusion

Throughout this book we've learned what cannabis is and how it works with our body's endocannabinoid system to treat a variety of ailments ranging from neurological diseases, cancer, stress, anxiety and a number of other conditions.

We've also touched on:
- *Cannabinoids and the difference between endo and Phyto cannabinoids*
- *The different species of cannabis and their therapeutic effects*
- *Titration & dosing, delivery methods, concentrations & tolerance*
- *Set & Setting*
- *Terpenes*
- *The "Entourage Effect"*
- *Opioids vs. Medicinal Cannabis*
- *A few of the more popular cannabinoids*
- *Specific things to consider while using cannabis*
- *Specifically, how various diseases and ailments can be treated with medicinal cannabis*

Although cannabis is something that ancient cultures have been using medicinally since 500 B.C., we are only now just starting to really learn more about this amazing plant and the many benefits that it provides us.

It's important to keep an open perspective on things and learn from our past in the sense that our viewpoints can change through a variety of different lenses such as those of moral, political, religious and cultural perspectives.

Hopefully this book has served as a good introduction into how cannabis is changing the way we look at and treat a variety of different medical conditions.

Although there is still much more to learn and many more clinical trials to be done, cannabis is showing amazing promise in regards to its medicinal use and the various life enhancing benefits that it provides.

Other Books By The Author

The Medicinal Cannabis Journal – A personal cannabis journal that helps you to track the products your using, symptom relief, which strains work best with your body, dosages, methods of administration and tracking additional cannabinoids.

Follow me on Instagram

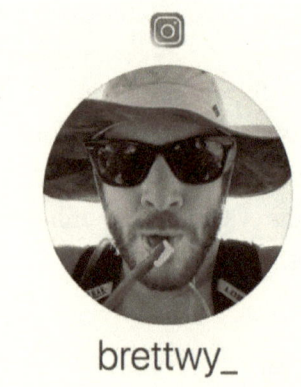

brettwy_

One Last Thing...

If you enjoyed reading this book and found it useful, I'd be extremely grateful if you gave me a review on Amazon.

The comments from my readers will help me to use the feedback and additional information to update the book and learn more about additional topics people would like to hear more of.

I personally read each review and I appreciate your support!

Works Cited

https://adaa.org/about-adaa/press-room/facts-statistics

https://www.anred.com/stats.html

https://apothecarium.com/blog/nevada/2018/5/14/cannabis-and-glaucoma

https://arthritis.ca/treatment/medication/medical-cannabis

https://www.arthritis.org/about-arthritis/understanding-arthritis/what-is-arthritis.php

https://www.arthritis.org/living-with-arthritis/pain-management/chronic-pain/arthritis-foundation-cbd-guidance-for-adults.php

https://www.atsdr.cdc.gov/substances/toxsubstance.asp?toxid=240

https://azcapitoltimes.com/news/2019/08/01/scottsdale-researcher-sues-u-s-government-over-quality-of-marijuana-for-studies/

https://www.cancer.gov/about-cancer/treatment/cam/hp/cannabis-pdq

https://www.cancer.org/cancer/cancer-basics/what-is-cancer.html

https://www.dementiacarecentral.com/parkinsons/treating/cbd/

https://www.drugabuse.gov/related-topics/trends-statistics/overdose-death-rates

https://www.drugfreeworld.org/drugfacts/ritalin.html#targetText=Ritalin%20is%20the%20common%20name,teens%20for%20its%20stimulant%20effects.

https://www.eaze.com/article/cannabis-for-nausea

https://www.farmapdx.com/the-ecs-at-a-glance/

http://files7.webydo.com/92/9209805/Uploaded-Files/5E9EC245-448E-17B2-C7CA-21C6BDC6852D.pdf

https://www.forbes.com/sites/abbierosner/2019/04/30/philanthropy-funds-cannabis-alzheimers-study/#2c6efa7c21bc

https://healthcareinamerica.us/cannabis-key-treating-ptsd-b4abf432215

https://www.healthline.com/health/CBD-reasons-it-doesnt-work#dosage-and-tolerance

https://www.healthline.com/health/depression/facts-statistics-infographic#1

https://www.healthline.com/health/epilepsy/facts-statistics-infographic#1

https://www.healthline.com/health/leading-causes-of-death

https://www.healthline.com/health/migraine/migraine-vs-headache

https://www.heylocannabis.com/post/what-are-terpenes

https://jamanetwork.com/journals/jama/article-abstract/338934?redirect=true

https://www.leafly.com/news/cannabis-101/terpenes-the-flavors-of-cannabis-aromatherapy

https://www.leafly.com/news/cannabis-101/factors-that-affect-your-cannabis-high

https://www.leafly.com/news/cannabis-101/cannabis-entourage-effect-why-thc-and-cbd-only-medicines-arent-g

https://www.leafly.com/news/cannabis-101/what-is-cbg-cannabinoid

https://www.leafly.com/news/cannabis-101/what-is-rick-simpson-oil

https://www.leafly.com/news/health/cannabis-and-arthritis

https://www.leafly.com/news/health/medical-marijuana-for-anorexia-treatment

https://www.mayoclinic.org/diseases-conditions/post-traumatic-stress-disorder/symptoms-causes/syc-20355967

https://migraine.com/migraine-treatment/natural-remedies/marijuana/

https://www.nationalmssociety.org/Treating-MS/Complementary-Alternative-Medicines/Marijuana/Marijuana-FAQs

https://www.nature.com/articles/nrd1495

https://www.ncbi.nlm.nih.gov/pmc/articles/PMC4171598/

https://www.ncbi.nlm.nih.gov/pmc/articles/PMC4588070/

https://www.ncbi.nlm.nih.gov/pubmed/?term=cannabis+nausea

https://www.ncbi.nlm.nih.gov/pubmed/25024327

https://www.ncbi.nlm.nih.gov/books/NBK224386/

https://www.ncbi.nlm.nih.gov/books/NBK224391/

http://pharmrev.aspetjournals.org/content/58/3/389.short

Pil Publications International, Ltd. Medical Marijuana – What You Need To Know. Favorite Brand Name Recipes, Vol. 1 No. 26, May 7, 2019.

https://psychcentral.com/blog/medical-marijuana-for-depression-bipolar-disorder-anxiety-mental-illness-can-it-help/

https://www.psycom.net/anxiety-depression-difference

https://www.psycom.net/eating-disorders/anorexia/

https://www.ptsd.va.gov/understand/common/common_adults.asp

https://www.sciencedirect.com/science/article/pii/S1525505013004629

https://www.sleepadvisor.org/sleep-statistics/

https://www.sleepfoundation.org/insomnia/what-insomnia

https://www.thegrowthop.com/cannabis-health/thcv-powerful-appetite-suppressing-cannabinoid

https://www.thegrowthop.com/cannabis-health/whats-the-difference-between-marijuana-cbd-and-hemp-cbd

https://thesleepdoctor.com/2018/11/27/thinking-about-using-cannabis-for-sleep-here-are-some-things-to-know/

https://www.theroc.us/researchli-brary/The%20role%20of%20the%20endocanna-binoid%20system%20in%20eating%20disorders-%20pharmacological%20implications.pdf

https://www.trulieve.com/blog/the-therapeutic-benefits-of-medicating-with-delta-8-thc?lo-cale=en

https://www.uclahealth.org/cannabis/human-en-docannabinoid-system

https://www.webmd.com/a-to-z-guides/medical-marijuana-faq

https://www.webmd.com/eye-health/glaucoma-eyes#1

https://www.webmd.com/migraines-head-aches/under-counter-treatment-migraines#1

https://www.webmd.com/multiple-sclerosis/mul-tiple-sclerosis-medical-marijuana#1

https://www.webmd.com/mental-health/what-are-treatments-for-posttraumatic-stress-disorder#1

https://www.webmd.com/women/pms/what-is-pms#2

https://www.westword.com/marijuana/why-a-federally-licensed-marijuana-researcher-is-suing-the-dea-11425543

https://www.wired.com/story/cannabis-science-entourage-effect/

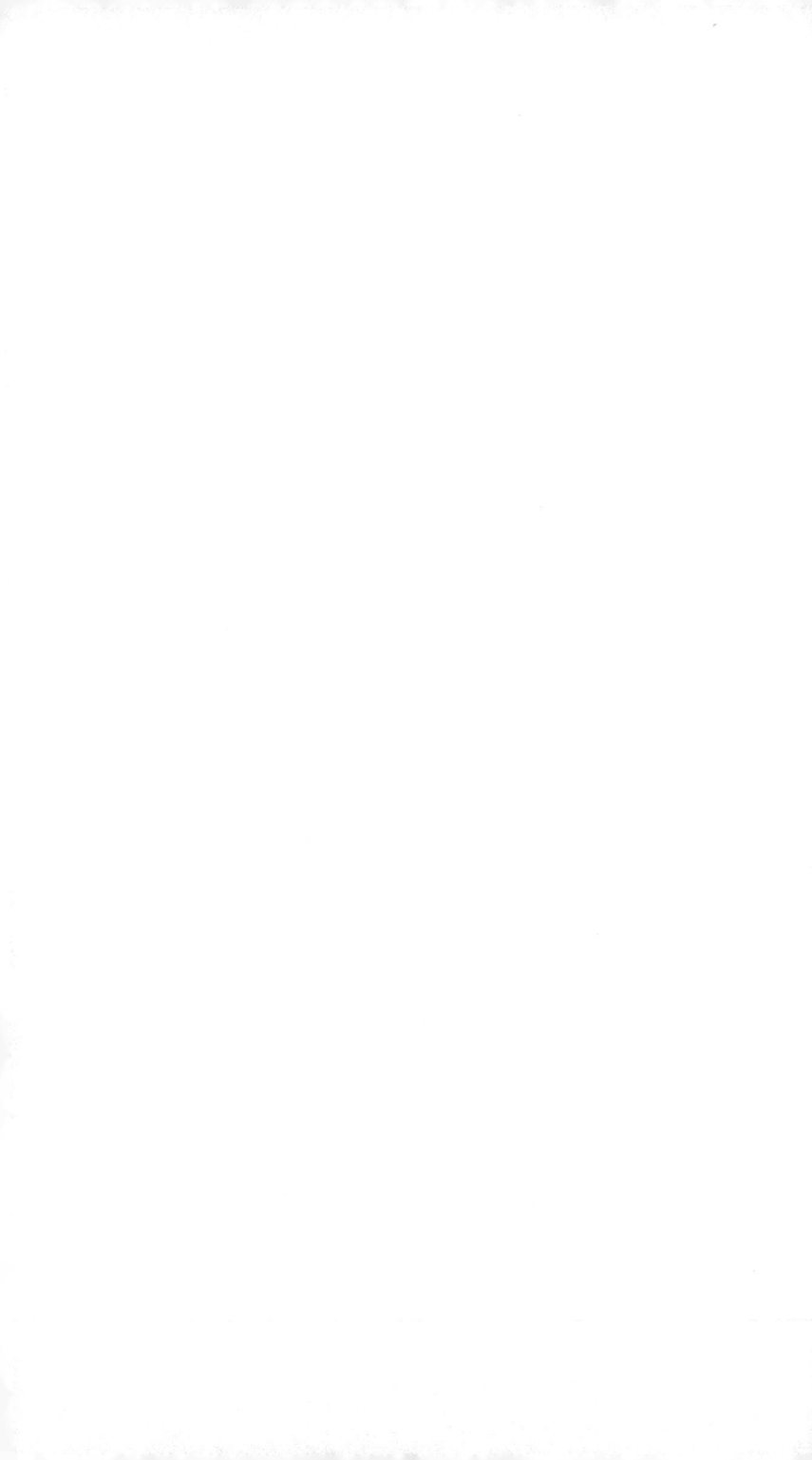